THE NEGATIVE CALORIE GUIDE

Lose Fat Without The Hunger And Reclaim Your Health

Carmen Donovan

Disclaimer

Contents

Introduction

Discover the Negative Calorie Diet

What is the first thing that comes to your mind when you hear the word 'diet?' Maybe starving, restricting your food intake, and even going hungry for hours, right? Well, all this is about to change now.

Yes, this eBook will change the way you look at diet and losing weight. You will discover foods that are low in calories, yet give you the daily required amount of vitamins, minerals and other nutrients.

Foods included in the negative calorie diet basically reduce your cravings for sweets and other unhealthy snacks. Basically the negative calorie diet keeps your energy levels steady so you don't become too hungry or fatigued soon. Perhaps the biggest advantage is that negative calorie foods boost your metabolic rate, burn calories and help you lose weight.

Broccoli, apple, celery and strawberries contain negative calories, i.e. they help burn more calories than the actual calorie content of the food itself. Eating a 5 calorie celery stick can help your body burn 100 calories which means you lose 95 calories from body fat.

Doesn't this sound interesting? Well, continue reading to find out more about negative calorie foods, how they work and the benefits of eating them. Also don't forget to check out the recipe section to know how you can include these fat burning foods into your lifestyle and lose weight in a healthy way.

Caution:

While this short guide is written to provide general information and advice, it cannot be used as a substitute for professional medical advice. Please consult your doctor before beginning any form of diet or weight loss program. Also, we encourage that elderly, pregnant women and anyone with any specific health condition or allergy seek help from a qualified healthcare provider before starting the negative calorie diet program.

If you're on medication or want to increase your physical activity, please consult your doctor. Your safety is of utmost importance.

Chapter One: What Are Negative Calories and How Do They Help With Weight Loss

To lose weight, you need to burn more calories than what you consume and here's where negative calorie foods come in handy. As stated earlier, negative calorie foods allow your body to burn or use more calories than the food actually contains.

For example: Your body might burn 100 calories to digest a 5 calorie piece of celery which means you achieve a net loss of 95 calories from your body fat. If you consider this equation, the more negative calorie foods you eat, the more weight you can lose.

How Does Negative Calorie Work?

All nutrients including carbohydrates, protein, vitamins and minerals have a calorie value. If you don't consume the amount of calories you eat, the excess is stored as fat leading to obesity and weight gain.

The best part about negative calorie foods is that they contain sufficient nutrition to keep you fit and healthy. That's right. You won't end up with nutrition deficiencies while following the negative calorie diet.

The other advantage is that negative calorie foods allow you to burn more calories than you eat, so you actually create a calorie deficit and lose weight.

It would be helpful to understand how your body digests food before we go into the details of negative calorie foods.

Digestion is a complex process. A series of physical and chemical changes take place inside your body before the food you eat can be absorbed by your body. When you eat something, the physical chewing process in your mouth and mechanical digestion in the stomach breaks down large pieces of food into smaller, manageable pieces.

The chemical digestion of the food also starts in the stomach where the food is mixed with stomach enzymes and gastric juices. After a couple of hours (depending on the type of food you eat), your food arrives in the small intestine and this is where the absorption and assimilation process takes place. Simply put, the glucose, fatty acids and amino acids broken down in the earlier steps are sucked up by your blood stream and distributed to different cells in your body.

Interestingly, an apple a day may or may not keep the doctor away, but this miraculous fruit surely can help you see some amazing results on the weighing scale. So does eating a bunch of celery and apples speed up your weight loss? Well, this is possible only if you eat them instead of saturated fat and refined sugar loaded stuff such as brownies and potato chips.

Remember, you can't devour a huge brownie and try to chase away the calories by eating plenty of celery sticks. You need to create a healthy eating plan and stick to it.

Replacing junk and other foods containing saturated fats and refined sugars with negative calorie foods can help you lose weight because you will reduce your overall calorie intake in a healthy way. Because these foods fill up the stomach and reduce satiety, you are less likely to grab that packet of crisps later on.

We want you to approach this diet differently than you have done in the past. Don't get stressed or upset. It's just simple. Read this guide a couple of times and go over the information closely. Also, talk to yourself and analyze your eating habits.

We want you to set challenging eating goals – remember, this diet change is not about setting impossible goals, but more about bringing a positive change. Understanding the digestion and metabolism process is the most important part of understanding how negative calorie foods work.

You have heard about metabolism right – the rate at which your body burns calories? Well, when your body breaks down carbohydrates, protein and fat, chemical energy is released as heat. This heat actually is what we refer to as calories. Foods that contain lots of energy for example fats have lots of calories. On the other hand, low energy foods have low calories.

As you know every person is different and so is their metabolism. You would know someone who eats without watching his meals for calorie amounts, yet he is slim. And then there are people with slow metabolism who aren't lucky as skinny people.

How do you speed up your metabolism? Yes, you've guessed it right. You can do this with the help of negative calorie foods. More specifically, you will be eating foods with very few calories, but your body won't sense the starvation. In fact, you would feel full and satisfied and at the same time, your body will continue to burn the excess stored fat.

What foods make up the negative calorie food list? Continue reading to find out more.

Chapter Two: Your Food Friends

Adding the following foods to your diet will help you see the inches melt away, due to their negative calorie properties. The more you add into your diet – or replace with – the more your health will improve.

<u>VEGGIES</u>

✓	Artichokes	✓	Celery
✓	Corn	✓	Mushrooms
✓	Asparagus	✓	Chives
✓	Cucumbers	✓	Onions
✓	Green beans	✓	Squash
✓	Dill pickles	✓	Parsley leaves
✓	Broccoli	✓	Tomato
✓	Eggplant	✓	Turnips
✓	Brussels sprouts	✓	Watercress
✓	Garlic	✓	Peas
✓	Cabbage	✓	Pumpkin
✓	Kale	✓	Radishes
✓	Carrots	✓	Rhubarb
✓	Leeks	✓	Scallions
✓	Cauliflower	✓	Shallots
✓	Lettuce	✓	Spinach

FRUITS

- ✓ Apples
- ✓ Kiwi
- ✓ Apricots
- ✓ Lemons
- ✓ Blackberries
- ✓ Mangoes
- ✓ Blueberries
- ✓ Nectarines
- ✓ Cantaloupe
- ✓ Oranges
- ✓ Cherries
- ✓ Papaya
- ✓ Cranberries

- ✓ Peaches
- ✓ Currants
- ✓ Pears
- ✓ Figs
- ✓ Pineapple
- ✓ Grapefruit
- ✓ Pomegranates
- ✓ Grapes
- ✓ Prunes
- ✓ Raspberries
- ✓ Strawberries
- ✓ Tangerines
- ✓ Watermelon

Chapter Three: Breakfast Recipes

Wonder what you can have for breakfast? Here are some amazing breakfast recipes you can try every morning to kick start your metabolism. Never skimp on breakfast as it is the most important meal of your day. We've rounded up our favorite breakfast options less than 300 calories to start your day right. When you're preparing your breakfast, you know what's going in so there are no secret calories or sugars to worry about.

1. Egg and Spinach Bowl

✓ This recipe provides 84 calories in each serving and approximately 11 grams of protein, 2 g of fat and 6 g of carbohydrates.

You will need:

- 1 whole egg

- 8 egg whites

- 1 cup baby spinach, you can chopped into small pieces

- ½ cup tomatoes, diced

- ¼ cup fat-free feta cheese

- black pepper and kosher salt to taste

Directions:

✓ Preheat oven to 350 degrees. Meanwhile combine all ingredients in a large mixing bowl and line four '½ cup' ramekins with cooking spray. Divide the egg and vegetable mixture evenly into 4 bowls and bake for 20 minutes or until eggs puff. Serve hot.

2. Avocado Toast

✓ This recipe yields 6 servings (one serving includes 1 tbsp avocado spread and 1 slice of toast). Calories 140, 6 g fat, 17 g carbohydrates and 5 g protein.

You will need:

- 6 slices whole wheat bread

- 1 ripe avocado

- 1 tsp balsamic vinegar

- 1 tsp extra virgin olive oil

- ¼ tsp crushed red pepper flakes

- Sea salt and black pepper to taste

Directions:

✓ Mix all ingredients except wheat slices in a food processor and blend until smooth. Toast bread and spread 1 tbsp avocado spread. You can sprinkle additional red pepper flakes if desired.

3. Cranberry and Raspberry Smoothie

✓ This vitamin C packed smoothie is an ideal start for your day. One serving provides 17g carbohydrates, 4 g proteins and 2g fat.

You will need:

- 200 ml cranberry juice

- 175g frozen raspberry

- 100 ml fat free milk

- 200 ml low-fat yogurt

- 1 tbsp caster sugar

Directions:

✓ Place all ingredients in a blender and pulse until smooth. Serve chilled topped with fresh mint leaves.

4. Perfect Porridge

✓ If you're looking to start your day in a healthy way, this recipe is one you should go for. Nutrition per serving: 25g carbohydrates, 10g protein and 5g fat. Total calories: 175.

You will need:

- 50g porridge oats

- 350 ml milk

- Water

Directions:

✓ Bring water to boil in a saucepan and simmer oats for about 4 to 5 minutes. Keep stirring from time to time. Once cooked, mix the oats with milk and pour into a large bowl. Drizzle raw honey and enjoy.

5. Asparagus and Eggs

✓ This classic recipe makes 4 servings. A single serving provides 12g carbohydrates, 12 g protein and 10g fat. Total calories: 186.

You will need:

- 4 eggs

- 50g breadcrumbs (dry)

- 16 to 20 asparagus spears

- Red chili and paprika to taste

- 1 tbsp olive oil

Directions:

✓ Heat olive oil and fry breadcrumbs until golden. Season with chili and paprika and allow the mixture to cool. Cook asparagus in boiling salt water until tender. Meanwhile boil the eggs and put them into 4 plates. Divide asparagus between the plates, sprinkle the crumbs and serve hot.

6. Tomato and Ham Omelet

✓ This 200 calorie recipe serves two and provides 12g fat, 5g carbohydrates and 21g protein in each serving.

You will need:

- 2 whole eggs
- 3 egg whites
- 1 red pepper finely chopped
- 2 spring onions finely chopped – separate green and white parts
- Extra lean ham, shredded
- 25g reduced fat cheddar cheese
- 1 – 2 tomatoes chopped
- One whole wheat toast (optional)
- 1 tsp olive oil

Directions:

✓ Mix the eggs and egg whites and set aside. Meanwhile sauté white part of the spring onion and pour in the eggs. Cook over medium heat until eggs are completely set.

✓ Sprinkle ham and cheese and continue cooking. Serve hot with green part of the spring onion and chopped tomatoes sprinkled on top.

7. Cinnamon Porridge

✓ This super healthy makes 4 servings. Each serving is 266 calories and provides 53g carbohydrates, 2g fat and 12g protein.

You will need:

- 3 bananas sliced

- 400g strawberries hulled and halved

- 150g natural yogurt

- ½ tsp cinnamon powder

- 100g porridge oats

- 450 ml skimmed milk

- 4 tsp sugar

Directions:

✓ Mix oats, milk, sugar and half the amount of sliced bananas in a saucepan and bring the mixture to boil. Lower the heat and continue cooking for an additional 4 to 5 minutes.

✓ Divide the mixture between 4 bowls and toss in the remaining bananas, strawberries and a teaspoon of yogurt. Sprinkle cinnamon powder and serve hot.

8. Berry Blast Smoothie

✓ This 123 calorie smoothie recipe provides 29g carbohydrates, 2g protein and 0g fat.

You will need:

- 1 small ripe banana

- 140g mixed berries – blueberries, blackberries, raspberries and strawberries

- Raw honey (optional)

Directions:

✓ Toss sliced bananas and berries into a food processor and pulse until smooth. You can pour in water to make the drink consistency you like. Drizzle raw honey on top and serve.

9. Cottage Cheese and Strawberries

✓ This 150 calorie breakfast serves one.

You will need:

- 1 cup non-fat cottage cheese

- 1 cup (approximately 80g) strawberries

- Cinnamon powder

Directions:

✓ Mix and toss both ingredients. Sprinkle cinnamon powder and enjoy a delicious treat.

10. Banana Berry Smoothie

✓ This recipe combines the ever popular banana with the healthy blueberry. Add this smoothie to your diet to boost your performance. Total calories: 143, 4g fat and 40g carbohydrates.

You will need:

- 150g fresh blueberries

- 1 Small Banana

- 220ml Pineapple Juice

Directions:

✓ Put all the ingredients into a blender and pulse until smooth. Easy, healthy and delicious. Enjoy!

Chapter Four: Lunch Recipes

Keeping your lunchtime eating regime on track is crucial if you want to lose weight. This section includes hearty recipes to help you make the most of your lunch break.

1. Vegetable and Bean Soup

✓ With 183 calories per serving, this soup is an ideal choice if you want to eat healthy and keep a close eye on your calories. Nutritional value: total fat 4g, protein 6g and carbohydrates 17g. Each serving size is approximately 1 ½ cups.

You will need:

- 2 carrots, peeled and sliced into thin 1" pieces
- 2 stalks celery, diced
- 1 sweet onion, diced
- 2 cloves garlic, minced
- 1 medium sweet potato, peeled and cut into 1" cubes
- 2 cups fresh green beans
- 4 cups vegetable broth, preferably low-sodium
- ¼ cup freshly chopped parsley
- 1 can diced tomatoes
- ½ tsp crushed red pepper flakes
- 2 cans black or pinto beans
- Kosher or sea salt to taste
- ½ tsp black pepper
- ½ tsp allspice
- 1 tsp paprika

Directions:

✓ Add all ingredients to a slow cooker and cook on low heat for about 8 hours or until the carrots are tender. This soup can be made ahead and taken to work.

2. Creamy Pasta Salad

✓ 1 cup pasta (single serving) provides 13g fat, 14g carbohydrates, and 5g protein and costs 190 calories.

You will need:

- 12 ounce penne pasta – cook according to package instructions

- 1 cup low-fat plain Greek yogurt

- ½ cup Pesto

- ¾ cup sun-dried tomatoes coarsely chopped

Directions:

✓ Combine yogurt with pesto and add to pasta. Toss well to coat. Sprinkle sundried tomatoes and garnish with fresh basil leaves.

3. Nutrient Dense Green Soup

✓ This super healthy recipe combines the goodness of kale, spinach and broccoli with the healing powers of coriander and turmeric. Each serving contains 182 calories, 14g carbohydrates, 5g fiber, 10g protein and 8g fat.

You will need:

- 500ml chicken stock

- 2 garlic cloves, sliced

- ½ tsp coriander (ground)

- 1 inch fresh ginger piece, sliced

- 1 tbsp sunflower oil

- 1 inch fresh turmeric root or ½ tsp turmeric powder

- Himalayan salt to taste

- 200g spinach, roughly sliced

- 100g kale, chopped

- Roughly chopped parsley, a bunch

- 1 lime, freshly juiced

✓ (*Ingredients make 2 servings)

Directions:

✓ Heat oil in a pan and sauté pinch of Himalayan salt, garlic cloves, sliced ginger, turmeric root, and coriander on medium heat for about 2 minutes. Now add spinach and mix well to coat in all the spices. Continue cooking for about 2 to 3 minutes.

✓ Add 400 ml stock and leave the soup to simmer for about 3 minutes.

✓ Next add kale, broccoli and fresh lime juice and continue to cook until the veggies are soft.

✓ Take the pan off the heat and pour the mixture into a blender. Pulse until the soup is smooth. Garnish with chopped parsley and serve hot.

4. Asparagus Soup

✓ Not many soups can beat the nutritional profile of this amazing vegetable soup prepared with a few simple ingredients. Each serving provides 8g fat, 4g carbohydrates, and 4g protein for the price of 101 calories!

You will need:

- 25g low-fat butter

- 350g asparagus spears – chop the stalks and reserve the tips. Woody ends should be discarded

- 3 finely sliced shallots

- 2 garlic cloves, crushed

- 700ml vegetable stock (preferably fresh)

- 2 large handfuls spinach

- Olive oil for drizzling (optional)

- A little vegetable oil

✓ *Ingredients make 4 servings

Directions:

✓ Heat butter in a large pan and fry the asparagus tips until soft. Now add the asparagus stalks, crushed garlic cloves and shallots and cook for an additional 5 to 10 minutes. Pour vegetable stock and toss in spinach leaves. Bring the soup to boil.

✓ Next, pour the mixture into a blender and pulse until smooth. Pour soup into bowls, drizzle with olive oil and serve hot.

5. Tomato and Carrot Soup

✓ This creamy soup recipe makes 8 generous servings.

✓ Nutritional Profile: 175 calories with 7g fat, 24g carbohydrates and 5g protein.

You will need:

- 2 red onions, chopped

- 2 celery sticks, chopped

- 250g potato, diced

- 1¼ kg carrot, sliced

- 750g cherry tomato

- 500g tomato passata

- 250ml whole milk

- 5 bay leaf (fresh or dried)

- 2 vegetable stock cubes

- 3 tbsp olive oil

- 1 tbsp granulated sugar

- 1 tbsp red wine vinegar

Directions:

✓ Heat olive oil in a large sauce pan and cook red onions and celery until softened. Now add sliced carrots and potatoes and cook for an additional 2 to 3 minutes.

✓ Add the remaining ingredients (except milk) and 1 liter water. Cover the sauce pan and simmer the soup for 25 to 30 minutes. Next, uncover the pan and simmer for an additional 20 minutes.

✓ Fish out the floating bay leaves and puree the soup with a hand blender. Next add milk and reheat gently before serving. You can make the soup and store it up to 2 to 3 days.

6. Chicken Soup

✓ This recipe yields about 10 servings. Nutritional Value 1 cup (single serving): 3g fat, 21g carbohydrates and 20g protein.

You will need:

- 2 chicken breasts fillets, skinless, cut into 1-2" cubes
- 2 ½ cup chicken broth, low-sodium and fat-free
- ½ cup diced onion
- 1 clove garlic, minced
- 1 can black beans, rinsed and drained*
- 1 can kidney beans, rinsed and drained
- 1 can diced green chili peppers
- 1 can diced tomatoes
- 1 cup fresh corn
- 1 tbsp fresh lemon juice
- ½ tsp black pepper
- Kosher or sea salt to taste
- 1 tbsp chili powder
- 1 tsp cumin (seeds)
- ½ cup cilantro, freshly chopped

✓ 1 can is 15 ounce.

Directions:

✓ Combine all ingredients in a slow cooker and cook for about 6 to 8 hours.

7. Potato and Carrot Soup

✓ Perfect for easy lunch, this soup can be prepared in less than 30 minutes. Each serving contains 3g protein, 19g carbohydrates and 4g fat for the price of 115 calories.

You will need:

- 1 red onion, chopped

- 1 potato, chopped

- 450g carrots, peeled and chopped

- 1200 ml chicken stock

- 1 tsp ground coriander

- 1 tbsp olive oil

Directions:

✓ Heat oil and cook onions for about 4 to 5 minutes or until soft. Toss in chopped potatoes and ground coriander and cook for an additional 2 minutes.

✓ Reduce heat and add chicken stock and carrots. Cover the sauce pan and cook the soup for about 20 minutes or until the carrots are tender. Pour the mixture into a blender and pulse until smooth. Return soup to the pan and reheat gently if needed. Serve hot.

8. Lentil and Carrot Soup

✓ You'll love this soup if you are in love with spicy foods. Each serving of this fabulous soup provides 17g carbohydrates, 4g protein and 1g fat and costs 92 calories.

You will need:

- 1 red onion, chopped

- 225g carrots, diced

- 75g red lentils

- 300ml orange juice

- 1 tsp cumin seeds

- 2 tsp coriander seeds

- 2 tbsp low-fat yogurt

- 600ml vegetable stock

- Freshly chopped coriander and pinch of paprika to garnish

Directions

✓ Crush cumin and coriander seeds and dry fry until brown. Add diced carrots, chopped onions, lentils, vegetable stock and orange juice to the pan and bring the mixture to the boil. Cover the pan and simmer for about 30 to 35 minutes until lentils are cooked and soft.

✓ Transfer the mixture to a food processor and blend until smooth. For best results, transfer and process the mixture in batches. Return soup to the pan and reheat gently.

✓ Pour the soup into individual serving bowls, sprinkle freshly chopped coriander, paprika and swirl the yogurt. Serve immediately.

9. Tomato Soup

✓ This soup tastes best with ripe and juicy tomatoes.

✓ Nutritional profile: Calories 123, 13g carbohydrates, 4g protein and 13g carbohydrates.

You will need:

- 1 kg ripe tomatoes cut into quarters

- 2 tsp tomato puree

- 1 medium red onion, chopped into small pieces

- 1 small carrot, chopped into small pieces

- 1 celery stick, chopped into small pieces

- 2 tbsp olive oil

- 1200ml vegetable stock made with 2 stock cubes and boiling water

- Bay leaf

- Pinch of sugar

Directions:

✓ Heat olive oil over medium heat and toss in chopped onions, celery and carrots. Mix the veggies together with a wooden spoon and cook until they are soft. Make sure the vegetables don't stick to the bottom of the pan.

✓ Add tomato puree and sprinkle a pinch of sugar and a little black pepper to the veggie mix. Tear a couple of bay leaves and throw them into the pan along with diced tomatoes.

✓ Stir the mixture and cook over low heat for 10 minutes. Slowly pour in the vegetable stock and cook the soup gently for 20 to 25 minutes. When tomatoes are soft and slushy, pour the mixture into a blender, fish out the bay leaf and turn the machine on.

✓ Pour the pureed soup back into the pan and add a pinch of salt and black pepper if you like. Serve chilled with some cream.

10. Artichoke Soup

✓ This low-fat soup provides 6g protein, 27g carbohydrates and 1g fat for the cost of 100 calories.

You will need:

- 200g raw vegetables chopped – you can use onions, celery and carrots

- 700 ml vegetable stock

- 300g potato, peeled and cubed

- 1 tbsp olive oil

- Fresh herbs – parsley, cilantro, oregano and thyme to garnish

Directions:

✓ Sauté raw vegetables in a little oil and then add the potatoes. Once potatoes begin to soften, pour in the stock and simmer for 10 to 15 minutes until the vegetables are tender.

✓ Blend the mixture until smooth, season with fresh herbs and serve hot. You can prepare the soup and freeze it up to one month.

Chapter Five: Dinner Recipes

The following dinner recipes are easy to make, delicious and most importantly, guilt free. Dinners often are the hardest part of a calorie controlled diet. Unless you are strict, it's quite easy to go overboard and eat more than you should.

This section includes dinner recipes that all come in under 300 calories. You can prepare a big batch and make portions for the week. Remember soups, salads included in the low calorie dinner recipes aren't just temporary diet substitutes. They are hearty, nutritious meals in their own right.

1. Crunchy Beans and Pepper Salad

This crunchy salad is greatly filling and quite appropriate as a healthy main course. Each serving costs 123 calories and provides 9 g fats.

You will need:

- 2 red peppers, halved and deseeded
- 2 yellow peppers, halved and deseeded
- 350g green beans, cooked
- 140g salad leaves

✓ For the dressing:

- 6tbsp olive oil
- 1tbsp freshly grated ginger
- 2tbsp balsamic vinegar
- 1tsp caster sugar

Directions:

✓ Preheat oven to 400 degrees Fahrenheit. Place the red and yellow peppers on a baking tray and roast them for about 20 to 30 minutes. Remove the tray and allow the peppers to cool. Remove the skin and roughly chop the peppers.

✓ Place peppers and green beans into a large bowl and pour over the dressing ingredients. Toss well and serve at room temperature.

2. Thai Mushroom and Chicken Broth

✓ This recipe serves 4 and is an ideal Thai treat for your taste buds.

✓ Nutritional Profile per serving: Calories 179, 6g carbohydrates, 25g protein and 6g fat.

You will need:

- 1000 ml (1 liter) chicken stock
- 1 tbsp Thai fish sauce
- 1 tbsp Thai red curry paste
- 2 tsp sugar
- 200g chicken, cooked and shredded
- 100g mushrooms, sliced
- 2 tbsp fresh lime juice
- 1 spring onion sliced – white and green part separated

Directions:

✓ Pour the stock into a large saucepan and add fish sauce, curry paste, fresh lime juice and sugar. Bring to boil and then add spring onion whites and mushrooms. Simmer for about 2 minutes.

✓ Stir in the chicken and spring onion greens. Heat thoroughly and then serve in individual bowls. You can serve with extra fish sauce and lime juice on the side so that people can adjust the taste to their liking.

3. Mint and Cucumber Salad

✓ This Thai inspired salad is super healthy and low calorie.

✓ Nutritional profile: Calories per serving 15, 3g carbohydrates, 1g protein and 0g fat.

You will need:

- 2 limes – cut out thin segments
- 1 large cucumber, peeled and finely sliced
- 1 tbsp white wine vinegar
- 1 small chili, finely sliced
- ½ tbsp sugar
- Fresh mint leaves

Directions:

✓ Place lime slices and half of the cucumber slices in a bowl and add vinegar and sugar. Cover and leave the bowl in the fridge overnight. Before serving, add remaining cucumber slices, sliced chili and toss together. Season with salt and vinegar if you like and sprinkle fresh mint leaves.

4. Squash Soup

✓ This recipe works for every occasion. You can skip the sherry if making soup for children.

✓ Nutritional profile: 183 calories per serving, 26g carbohydrates, 5g fiber and 4g protein.

You will need:

- 1kg butternut squash peeled. Remove the seeds and chop into small pieces

- 1 large onion, halved

- 4 tbsp dry sherry

- 600ml hot vegetable stock

- 2 tbsp olive oil

Directions:

✓ Fry the onions until softened. Next add the squash and sherry and sizzle for about 2 to 3 minutes.

✓ Pour in the vegetable stock and cover and simmer until the squash is tender. Pour the mixture into a food processer and blend until smooth. This soup can be kept in the fridge for a couple of days. When ready to eat, reheat the soup and serve with seed bread croutons.

5. Greek Lamb Salad

✓ This Greek dish is nothing less than a satisfying dinner.

✓ Nutritional profile: 306 calories per serving, 17g fat, 5g carbohydrates and 32g protein. This recipe makes 4 servings.

You will need:

- 140g lean lamb steaks x 4

- 3 large tomatoes, cut into large chunks

- ½ cucumber, cut into small chunks

- 50g pitted black olives

- 75g crumbled feta

- ½ tbsp lemon juice

- 1 tbsp olive oil

- ½ tsp oregano, dried

- Mint leaves

- Salt and black pepper, to taste

Directions:

✓ Mix dried oregano, lemon juice, salt, olive oil and black pepper in a large bowl. Add the lamb steaks and turn around to coat. Set the grill to its hottest setting and cook the lamb steaks until done to your liking. Transfer to a plate and cover loosely with foil. Let the steaks rest for 3 to 5 minutes and then cut thick slices.

✓ Divide the steaks between 4 plates and add tomatoes, cucumber and olives. Top with small chunks of feta, scatter mint leaves and then serve.

6. Leek and Bacon Soup

✓ Nutritional profile: 175 calories per serving, 6g protein, 15g carbohydrates and 11g fat. This recipe serves 4 to 6.

You will need:

- 400g leek, washed and sliced
- 3 medium potatoes, peeled and diced
- 1400 ml vegetable stock
- 3 rashers streaky bacon, chopped
- 1 red onion, chopped
- 25g butter
- 140 ml low fat cream

Directions:

✓ Melt the butter in a large pan and fry the onions and bacon until they turn golden. Toss in the potatoes and leeks, mix well and lower the heat. Cook gently for 5 minutes, season and then pour in the stock.

✓ Cover the pan and bring the mixture to a boil. Simmer for about 20 minutes until the veggies are soft.

✓ Allow the mixture to cool and then blend in a food processor until it is smooth. Return the soup to the pan, pour in the cream and mix well. Serve hot.

7. Crusted Salmon

✓ Nutritional profile: 315 calories per serving, 17g protein, 33g carbohydrates and 15g fat. This recipe serves 4.

You will need:

- 4 skinless salmon fillet
- ½ lemon, cut into wedges
- 500g baby potatoes
- 25g butter
- 4 tbsp fresh (white) breadcrumbs
- 1 ½ tsp peppercorns, coarsely ground
- Cooked broccoli, green onions
- Fresh thyme

Directions:

✓ Place potatoes in a large pan of salted water. Cover and bring to boil. Simmer for 15 minutes until potatoes are cooked. Meanwhile combine lemon zest, butter and peppercorns.

✓ Roast salmon fillet and sprinkle 1 tbsp of crumbs. Bake salmon at 200 degrees Fahrenheit for 8 to 10 minutes until it is fully cooked.

✓ When potatoes are cooked, drain and crush lightly. Add butter and seasoning and serve with roasted salmon, broccoli and spring greens.

8. Avocado and Chicken Salad

✓ Nutritional Profile: 350 calories per serving, 34g protein, 18g carbohydrates and 19g fat. This recipe serves 2.

You will need:

- 175g cooked chicken

- 1 avocado, stoned, peeled and sliced

- 85g blueberries

- 85g bag baby salad leaf mix

- 125g fresh baby broad beans – boiled until tender

- 1 large beetroot, cooked and finely chopped

- 1 garlic clove, finely chopped

- 1 tbsp extra virgin rapeseed oil

- 2 tsp balsamic vinegar

Directions:

✓ Mash blueberries with rapeseed oil, vinegar and black pepper in a large bowl and toss in crushed garlic. Now add in the beans, avocado, beetroot, mixed salad leaf and chicken. Toss but take care not to go overboard or the salad will turn pink! Serve in shallow plates.

9. Mediterranean Fish Soup

✓ Nutritional profile: 164 calories per serving, 23g protein, 4g fat and 9g carbohydrates.

You will need:

- 450 ml fish stock

- 2 courgette, finely sliced

- 1 fennel bulb, finely sliced

- 500g tomato and basil pasta sauce

- 450g hoki fillet

- 1 tsp chipotle chili

- Fresh basil leaves

Directions:

✓ Put pasta sauce and stock in a large sauce pan. Simmer and bring the mixture to the boil. Add courgette and fennel and simmer for 2 minutes.

✓ Next cut the hoki fillet into 4 cm small pieces. Add the fish fillet to the soup and cook for about 2 to 3 minutes over low heat. Remember, you need to stir the soup gently or the fish will break. Toss in basil leaves and adjust the seasoning. Pour into individual bowls and then serve.

10. Smoked Salmon with Poppy

✓ Nutritional profile: 99 calories per serving, 13g protein, 4g fat and 2g carbohydrates.

You will need:

- 300g smoked salmon
- 85g radish, finely sliced
- 1 tbsp poppy seed, lightly toasted
- 2 orange – zest of both and juice of 1
- 2 tsp red wine vinegar
- 2 tsp olive oil
- ½ tsp sesame oil
- 3 spring onion, finely sliced

Directions:

✓ Whisk toasted poppy seeds with orange zest, orange juice, black pepper, salt, vinegar and oils. This will be your salad dressing.

✓ Mix salmon slices with radish and spring onions. Drizzle the dressing generously and toss gently to mix all ingredients. Spread the salad over a large plate and scatter any remaining radishes and spring onions. Enjoy the healthy treat.

Chapter Six: Vegetarian and Vegan Recipes

Finding inspiration for vegan and vegetarian cooking isn't as difficult as people might think. Here are some incredibly satisfying and tasty low calorie vegan recipes that can make your day.

1. Vegetarian Taco Salad

✓ This salad can be quickly assembled at lunch or dinner.

✓ Nutritional profile: 350 calories per serving (1 ½ cups each), 17g fat, 48g carbohydrates and 14g protein. The recipe makes about 6 servings.

You will need:

- 2 tbsp extra-virgin olive oil
- 1 large red onion, chopped
- 1 ½ cup fresh corn kernels
- 4 large tomatoes
- 1 ½ cup cooked brown rice
- 1 can pinto beans, rinsed
- 1 tbsp chili powder
- 1 ½ tsp dried oregano
- ¼ tsp salt, black pepper
- ½ cup fresh cilantro, chopped
- 1/3 cup salsa
- 2 cups romaine lettuce, shredded
- 2 ½ cups tortilla chips, coarsely crumbled
- Lime wedges (optional for garnish)

Directions:

✓ Heat oil in a large skillet over medium heat and cook onions and corn for 2 to 3 minutes. Add tomato paste to the pan along with beans, brown rice, chili powder, 1 tsp oregano and salt. Keep stirring frequency and cook the 'bean mixture' for about 5 minutes.

✓ Combine freshly chopped cilantro with salsa and remaining oregano in a medium bowl. Toss salad leaves with the bean mixture and pour the salsa dressing. Sprinkle crushed tortilla and lime wedges before serving.

2. White Bean Soup

✓ This simple yet rich white beans soup recipe makes about 8 servings (1 ½ cups). Nutritional profile: 258 calories, 4g fat, 14g protein and 42g carbohydrates.

You will need:

- 1 pound dried white beans, soaked overnight
- 2 tbsp extra-virgin olive oil
- 2 large red onions, finely chopped
- 2 celery stalks, finely chopped
- 2 large carrots, finely chopped
- Water
- 1tbsp tomato paste
- 2 tsp dried oregano
- 1 tsp salt
- 1/8 tsp cayenne pepper
- Salt and black pepper, to taste

Directions:

✓ Drain and cook white beans in a large pan until tender. Sauté onions, celery and carrots for 3 to 5 minutes and then add water, cooked beans, oregano, cayenne, salt and black pepper. Simmer until veggies are tender. Adjust seasoning and serve.

3. Roasted coriander and cauliflower

✓ This recipe serves 4. Nutritional profile: 118 calories per serving, 7g fat, 9g carbohydrates and 5g protein.

You will need:

- 500g cauliflower, cut into florets

- 1 tsp ground coriander

- 2 red onions (slice into thick wedges)

- 2 tbsp olive oil

- Handful fresh coriander

Directions:

✓ Preheat oven to 220 degrees Celsius. In a roasting pan, toss cauliflower, sliced onions, ground coriander, and olive oil with some salt and pepper. Roast the veggies for 20 to 25 minutes and keep tossing occasionally. When vegetables start to brown, remove the pan, sprinkle fresh coriander and serve.

4. Falafels

✓ This recipe makes 6 servings. Nutritional profile: 105 calories, 6g fat, 5g protein and 8g carbohydrates.

You will need:

- 2 tbsp sunflower oil
- 1 small red onion, finely chopped
- 1 garlic clove, crushed
- 400g chickpeas, washed and drained
- 1 tsp ground cumin
- 1 tsp ground coriander
- Handful parsley, chopped,
- 1 egg, beaten

Directions:

✓ Heat 1 tbsp oil in a large pan and fry crushed garlic and chopped onions over a low heat for 4 to 5 minutes. Mash chickpeas until they are broken down and stir in the parsley and seasoning to taste. Add the beaten egg and mix the ingredients with your hands.

✓ Mould the mixture into balls and then flatten them to make patties. Heat the remaining oil and fry the falafel. Serve with toasted pita bread or salad.

5. Tofu Kebabs

✓ This recipe serves 4. Nutritional profile: 178 calories per serving, 8g fat, 18g carbohydrates and 10g protein.

You will need:

- 300g firm smoked tofu, cut into cubes
- 1 courgette, peeled and sliced
- 1 red pepper, deseeded and diced
- 8 shallots, cooked in boiling water
- 8 small new potatoes, cooked in boiling water
- 1 tbsp raw honey
- 1 tbsp wholegrain mustard
- 2 tbsp tomato puree
- 2 tbsp light soy sauce
- 1 tbsp sunflower oil

Directions:

✓ Put tomato puree, soy sauce, oil, honey, mustard and seasoning in a large bowl and mix well. Toss the tofu in the mixture and set aside for 10 to 15 minutes.

✓ Thread the marinated tofu, peppers, courgette, shallots and potato on a skewer. Grill for 10 minutes turning the sides frequently. Once done, drizzle the remaining marinade and serve hot.

Chapter Seven:
Snacks and On-The-Go Eating

Fill your kitchen cabinet with these low calorie snacks that support your negative calorie diet program. These snacks are ideal during the toughest times, i.e. when you get that hunger pangs.

1. Handful of Almonds or Walnuts

✓ Eat 14 almonds or 8 walnuts and you can curb those cravings without hitting the 100 calorie mark.

2. 1 glass whey protein with water

✓ Whey protein perhaps is the easiest 'grab and go' source of essential amino acids. What's better is that it costs less than 100 calories.

3. 1 sweet potato, boiled (98 calories)

✓ If you want to keep your energy stores up without adding calories, add one boiled sweet potato to your diet.

4. 25g instant oatmeal

✓ This speedy snack costs less than 100 calories and provides constant energy for hours.

5. 1 boiled egg (approximately 78 calories)

6. 1 medium size banana – 100 calories

7. 200g papaya or 300g water melon

✓ These fruits are low in sodium and calories and satisfy your hunger with fewer calories

8. 1 cup broccoli – 25 calories

✓ 1 cup calorie requires up to 80 calories for digestion which means you can burn 55 calories by just eating it. If you don't like broccoli, go for celery or zucchini.

9. 1 cup banana smoothie

✓ Blend ¼ cup fat free yogurt with ½ banana and ice cubes. This refreshing drink is nutritious and costs 95 calories.

10. 1 cup chopped watercress that costs 34 calories

✓ Watercress is easy to add onto any meal, but it's also great as a snack. It looks good, tastes great and really packs a strong negative calorie effect.

Chapter Eight: Top Tips for Eating Out On a Negative Calorie Diet

It's not easy to dine out when you're keeping a close eye on your calorie count. However, this doesn't mean you refuse to go out with friends and family. The following tips can help you eat smart while dining out. After reading this section, you can dine out successfully without messing up your dieting plan.

1. Know what you want to eat

✓ Most restaurants these days have online menus and you can actually see what dishes they offer. Go for healthier options such grilled, salads, and vegetables sides. Also, avoid dishes with heavy, creamy and fattening sauces.

2. Have it your way

✓ It's always good to ask the server about the details of the meal. Sometimes you can modify the ingredients and choose low-fat or low-calorie options. Some restaurants allow you to change the portion size. Remember, as a paying customer, you shouldn't be afraid to make a special request. Ask if a particular dish can be baked rather than fried. If the ingredients are listed on the menu, the chef should be able to accommodate your needs.

3. Stay away from appetizers

✓ If you plan to eat out, you should stay away from the appetizers as they are usually loaded with fat. Remember, nothing comes free and freebies like chips and salsa can add up extra calories that you don't need.

4. Be Nutrition Savvy

✓ Your food can be your best friend or worst enemy depending on what you choose. Even if you choose healthy greens, beans, fruits, it's not going to help if you drown the salad with high-fat sauces and dressings. Pick low calorie dressings such as vinaigrettes; in fact even a generous squeeze of fresh lemon can work wonders.

5. Substitute high fat dishes with low-calorie options

✓ Substitute high calorie dishes such as beef with low calorie options such as brown rice, fresh fruits and steamed vegetables. You can have baked or boiled or roasted potatoes but skip the French fries. If you want to flavor a soup or salad, leave out cheeses and creams. Use pepper and chives instead.

Conclusion

✓ The food choices you make each day affect your health. That's right. What you eat decides how you will feel today, tomorrow and in the future. Eating right is an important part of leading a healthy lifestyle. If combined with physical activity, eating the right negative calorie foods can help you reach and maintain a healthy weight.

✓ What's better is that negative calorie foods give you the required nutrition (vitamins, minerals, protein and carbohydrates) and at the same time reduce your risk of chronic diseases.

✓ The nutrition contained in negative calorie foods can protect your cells from environmental damage and repair any damage that might occur at the cellular level. Vitamins and minerals as you can guess are crucial for support of your body's important physiological processes. Vitamin C, A and E in particular are powerful antioxidants and help protect your cells against toxins and free radical damage.

✓ Eating processed foods or those containing saturated fats is not at all good for your health and wellbeing. Numerous medical studies suggest that people who engage in unhealthy eating and unhealthy habits such as smoking, drinking and lack of physical activity are at an increased risk for developing serious medical complications.

✓ Most diets unfortunately are about the same thing – restricting calories. Of course you need to cut down calories to lose weight, but the secret to weight loss is not eating less, it's about eating right.

✓ Now that we have reached the end of this eBook, you should have a good idea about negative calorie foods and how they work. These nutritious foods provide you with the much needed nutrition and at the same time help burn fat and lose weight. Because negative calorie foods themselves are low calorie, you can add them to your dinner, lunch and breakfast recipes and kickoff a healthy eating plan.

✓ It's high time you have a thorough check of your shopping list and pantry. If you really want to be healthy, make sure your grocery list includes foods that have a negative caloric effect, i.e. they burn more calories than they contribute. You can always refer to the list of negative calorie foods if you need an inspiration for grocery shopping.

✓ Remember, once you have decided to change your eating habits, it's important that you stick with your lifestyle changes. Feel free to experiment with the recipes and here's hoping that you are on the road to healthy eating. Perhaps the best part about negative calorie foods is that they can help you lose pounds and build healthy habits that last a lifetime. So never give up!